My Boy, W

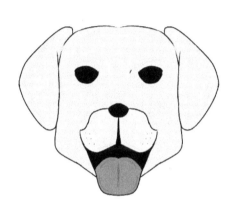
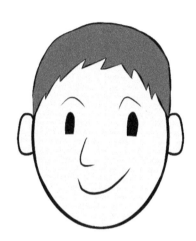

Written and Illustrated by

William J. Gibney
with
Dr. Laura A. Assaf

ISBN 978-1506-902-18-0 HCJ
ISBN 978-1506-900-97-1 PBK
ISBN 978-1506-906-65-2 EBK

LCCN 2021910486

November 2021

Published and Distributed by
First Edition Design Publishing, Inc.
P.O. Box 17646, Sarasota, FL 34276-3217
www.firsteditiondesignpublishing.com

To Dr. Emily Zier,
for changing the world one service dog at a time.

A note from Dr. Assaf

Though Will has been blessed by many angels who have crossed his path - from the brilliant and extraordinary doctors who knew what they were seeing and how to treat it, and the unconventional administrators who embraced Will and kept him in school despite his behavioral disruptions, to the inquisitive and passionate educators who saw him as a child who was meant to teach the rest of us about neurodiversity - it was not until Will was matched with Skilled Companion Toshi II that he began to produce antibodies in response to infections. Only then did he begin to demonstrate a typical or expected immune response.

Within three months of having Toshi at home, living life next to him, and sleeping in his bed at night, Will's immunological profile began to change, and so did his behavior. Will became more independent and mature as he started caring for another being instead of needing everyone else to care for him. The character gifts Will has - his kindness, perseverance, generosity of spirit, and empathy for others - were no longer overshadowed by the incongruent behaviors he demonstrated when his brain was inflamed.

For that reason, among countless others, proceeds from the sale of *My Boy, Will* will go to Canine Companions in gratitude for the gift that Toshi has been to Will and his entire family.

As so eloquently stated by Dean Koontz, Celebrity Supporter and Honorary National Board Member of Canine Companions,

"Once you have had a wonderful dog, a life without one, is a life diminished."

We hope you enjoy Will's story of how he was matched with Skilled Companion Toshi II, his superhero dog who wears a vest instead of a cape. I wrote the last few pages of the story to acknowledge how Will and Toshi have changed and inspired me and my clinical practice.

With unending gratitude to Canine Companions and our beloved Guilderland community for Will's health and recovery,

Laura A. Assaf, Psy.D.
Licensed Psychologist, but more importantly, Will's Mom 🩶

My boy, Will, is fun. My boy, Will, is smart. My boy, Will, loves to swing, play imagination, visit his friends, and travel the world. He loves gems and minerals, superheroes, dragons, and comic books. He is an artist, a musician, and a good friend.
That is when my boy, Will, is healthy.

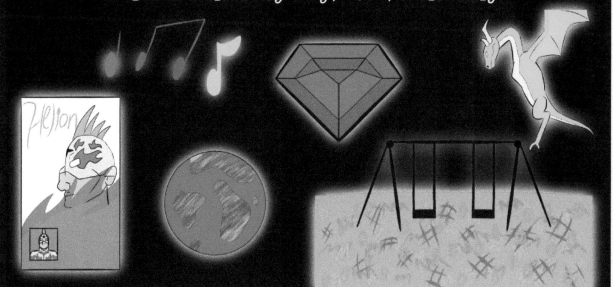

When my boy, Will, was sick, a change would come over his body. His cheeks would turn red. His eyes got wide and glassy. His body would twitch and tic and move in a strange way.

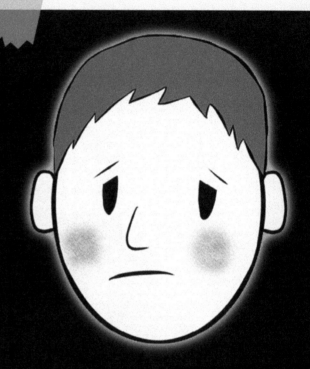

Will had to do things like pick at a bug bite until it bled, straighten all the shoes in the house, or gather all the straw wrappers from the floor in a restaurant.

In second grade, when he was infected, Will could not go into the cafeteria if there was fruit on the floor. When he was not well in fifth grade, Will could not enter his classroom if there were pencils on the floor.
There are always pencils on a classroom floor!

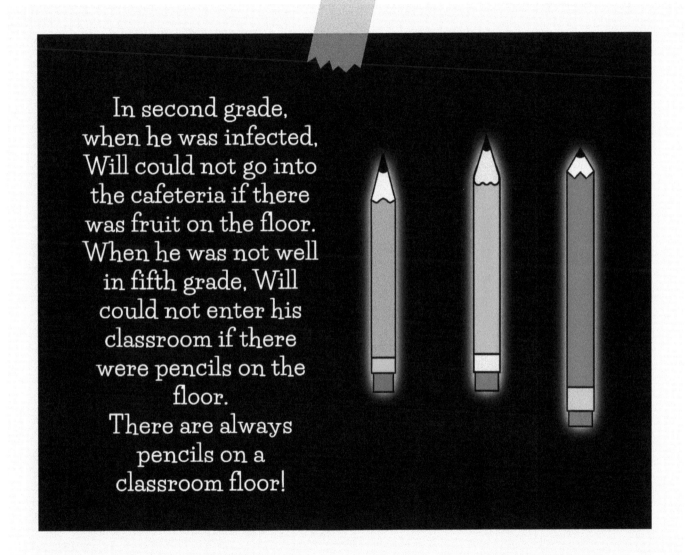

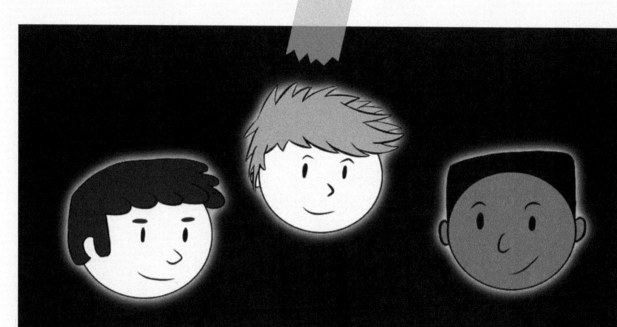

Since Will is such a cool kid, he had good friends who would run around and clean up the pencils so he would not get stuck in the doorway. But needing friends to do that can make a kid feel sad or weird.

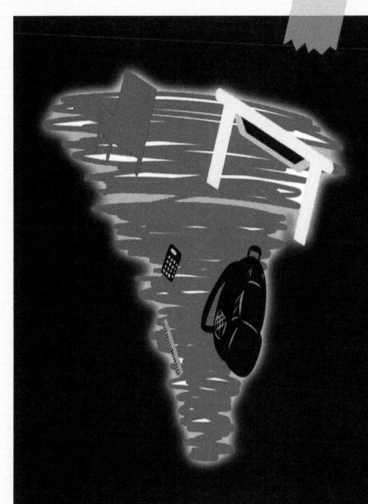

And then there were the things kids are not supposed to do in school, like tear down bulletin boards, or push desks or people when they are desperate to get out of the classroom but they don't even know why.
That used to happen to my boy, Will, too.

They tell me that Will has loved dogs since he was a baby. So it made sense that Will's mom would try to find him a dog to help him, especially when he was 11-years-old and he needed to spend a lot of time in the hospital, building a healthier body.

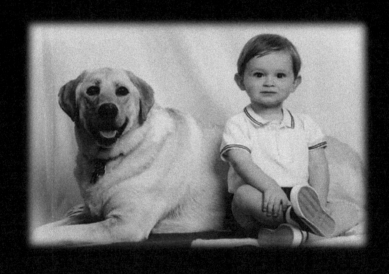

I met Will the summer after I finished my advanced training at Canine Companions and was waiting to see if my forever person was in that big group of humans that arrived to the training center. All the new people seemed nice, but nervous. There were adults and children in wheelchairs or walkers, and some other people whose disabilities or needs we dogs could not see.

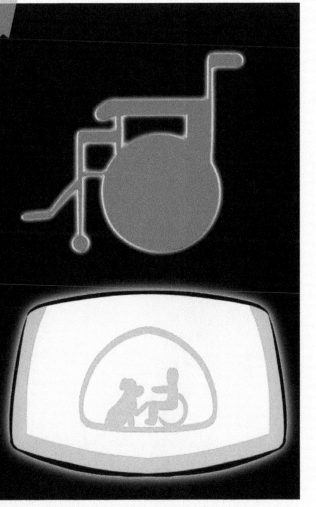

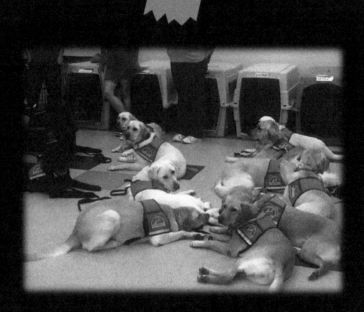

The first time I heard Will's voice was when he introduced himself to the group. He said, "Hi. I'm Will. I have PANS." Then Will's mom started talking. She said that Will's body is chronically (that's a big word, it means always) fighting infection, and often losing.

The infections inflame his brain (that sounded scary!) and make him think the same thought over and over again, or say the same word over and over again.

What what what what what what
what what what what what what
what what what what what what
wnat what what what what what
what what what what what what
what what what what what what
what what what what what wnat
what what whae what what what
what wnot what what what what

When he was infected, Will would feel afraid, or sad, or angry, or really hyper. Sometimes Will would forget what he learned in school, especially math and how to write like a big kid, and he would act much younger than he was.

2 + 2 = ?

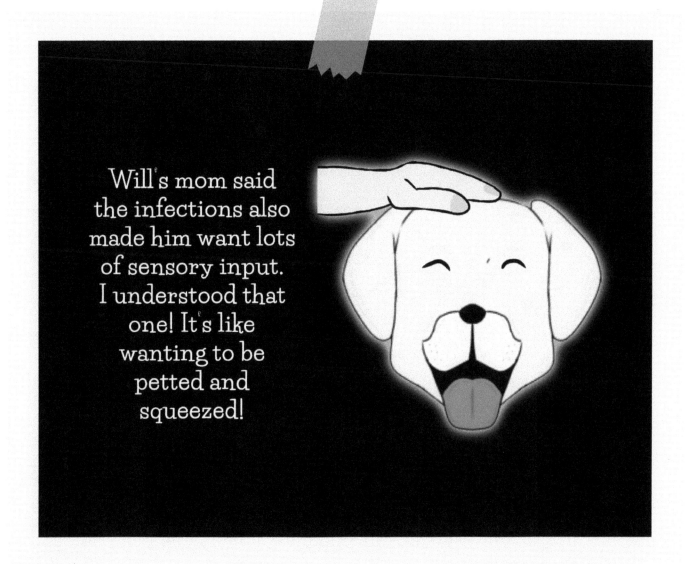

Will's mom said the infections also made him want lots of sensory input. I understood that one! It's like wanting to be petted and squeezed!

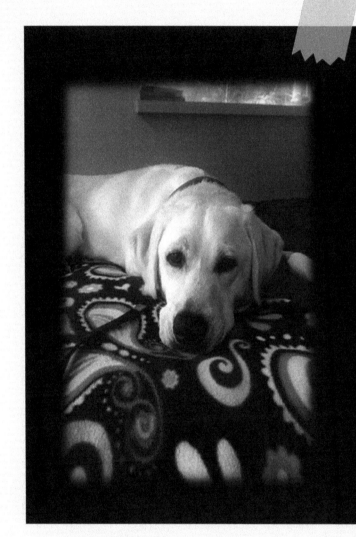

Will's mom said that Will was brave and strong and smart and an advocate. I knew that word meant someone who teaches others about something new or special or different, and helps others understand.
I really wanted to meet Will.

When the humans get trained at Canine Companions, they spend time with many different dogs. I watched Will and his mom working with my friends, Elena and Erickson, two great dogs, but not me. I did not understand why they were keeping us apart! I knew Will was meant for me. Why didn't they want me meet Will?

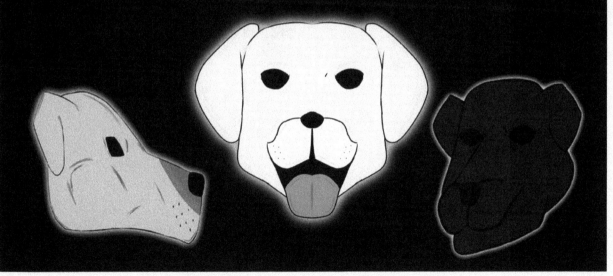

But then the moment came when I was out in the hallway, away from the group. One of the trainers called Will's mom out to join us, but they had Will stay in the group training room. What a tease! But Will's mom started petting me and telling me what a nice boy I was. She started to command me with, "Stand," and "Let's go!"

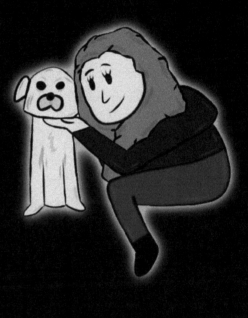

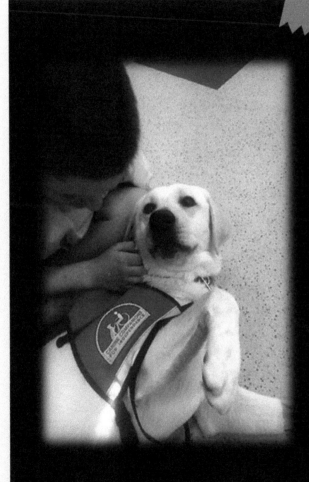

I wanted to impress Will's mom, but then the doors banged open and there he was! I was so distracted I stopped listening to Will's mom. I needed to get to that boy!
I wagged my tail and wiggled my butt as hard as I could. Will laughed and came right to me, and I covered him with wet kisses!

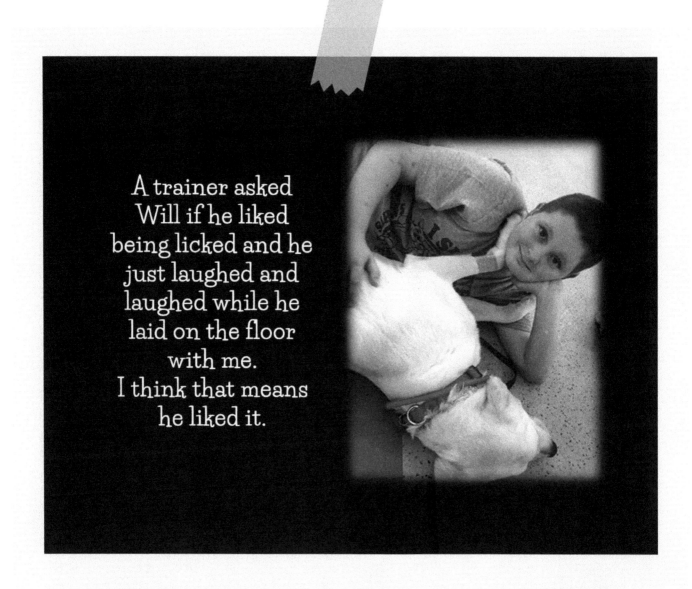

A trainer asked
Will if he liked
being licked and he
just laughed and
laughed while he
laid on the floor
with me.
I think that means
he liked it.

But then they made Will leave! He needed to "hurry" (that means to go outside and pee where you are told). Will hurries a lot. I heard his mom say that is part of his condition. Oh, I hoped I'd get to hurry with Will!

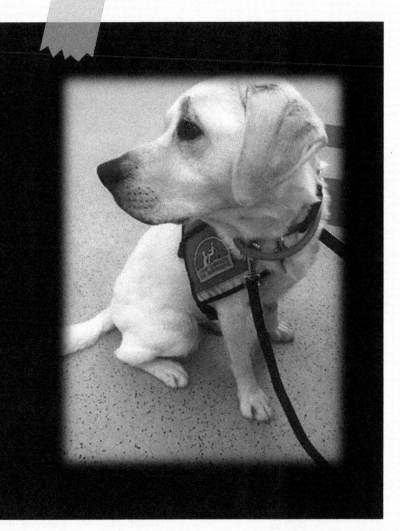

I watched Will bound down the hallway and didn't want to do my commands anymore. I wanted to be with Will! I heard his mother say that it was like I "imprinted" on Will, which was weird because that's what baby birds do when they first see an animal that is supposed to take care of them when they hatch. I'm no baby! I am going to be two years-old-soon. And a real working dog! But I did like watching Will with all his big energy and floppy movements.

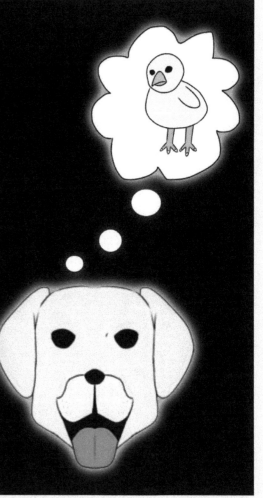

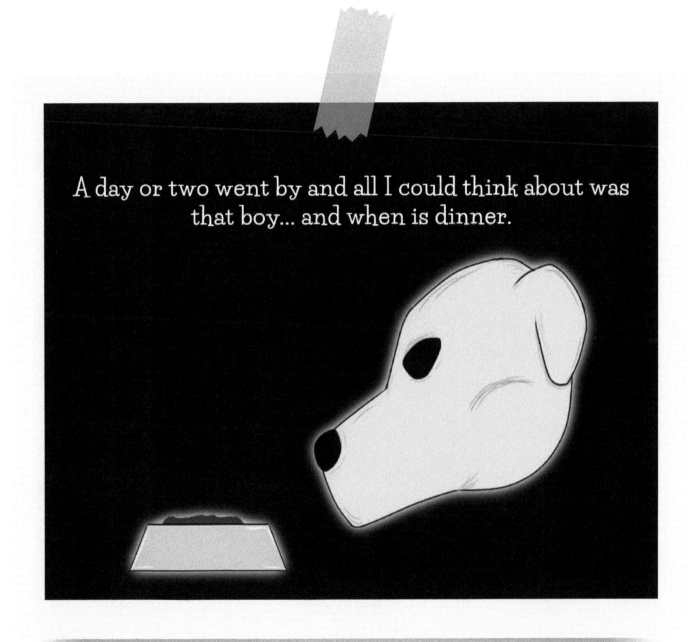

A day or two went by and all I could think about was that boy... and when is dinner.

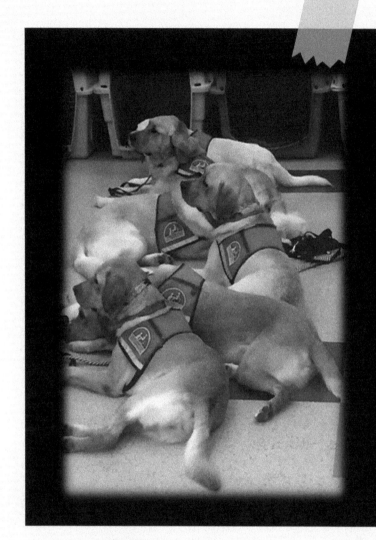

Then finally came match day. That is the moment we find out who we will be our forever human. I laid on the floor with all of my buddies and you could feel the excitement in the air.

I listened as two other dogs got matched, but I never took my eyes off Will. And then my trainer, Marissa, stood next to the board. She said, "Our next match is with our yellow lab-golden cross named Toshi II. Toshi is matching with...Will!" I jumped to my feet and trotted to my boy. He fell to the floor and covered me with hugs!

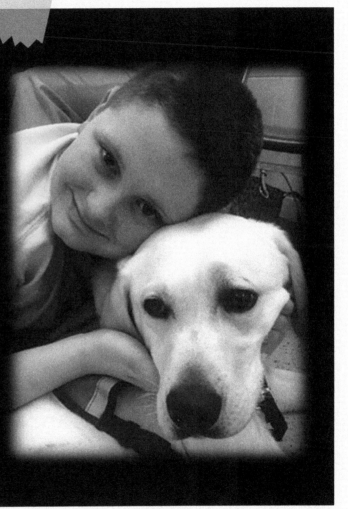

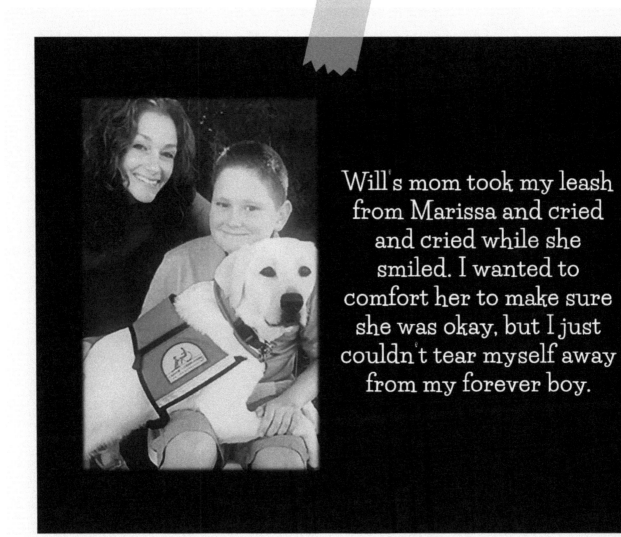

Will's mom took my leash from Marissa and cried and cried while she smiled. I wanted to comfort her to make sure she was okay, but I just couldn't tear myself away from my forever boy.

We spent the next 10 days of training getting to know each other and working hard! I learned that Will was not able to sit in one place for very long. He was always shifting and moving. He did better when he was drawing, often while lying on his stomach. Will needed lots of breaks from training, but his breaks got shorter and shorter when he had me to snuggle.

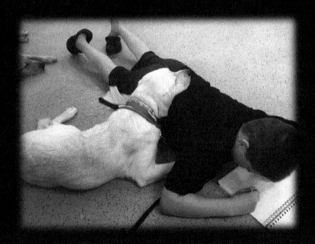

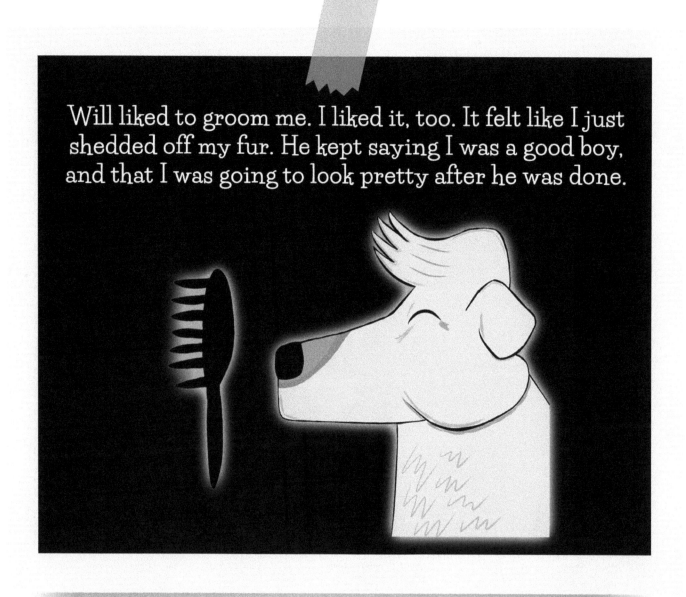

Will liked to groom me. I liked it, too. It felt like I just shedded off my fur. He kept saying I was a good boy, and that I was going to look pretty after he was done.

Soon graduation day came. I thought it was just the day I would get to go home with Will. I had no idea that before that happened, I would be re-united with Emily, my puppy raiser. Graduation day turned out to be the greatest day ever! It brought my two favorite humans together.

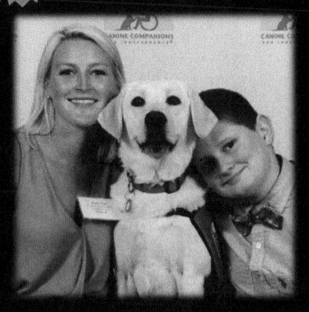

I knew Emily would love Will and that he would love her. I had to say goodbye to Emily, but she and Will promised to see each other again, and I knew they would keep their promise.

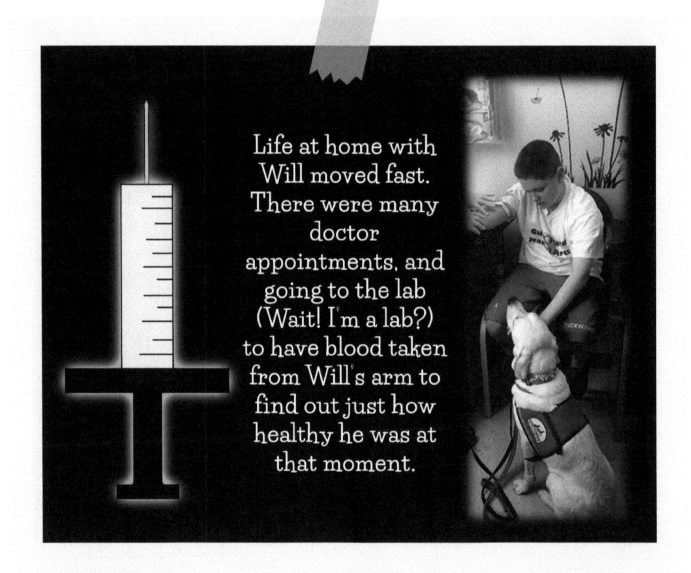

Life at home with Will moved fast. There were many doctor appointments, and going to the lab (Wait! I'm a lab?) to have blood taken from Will's arm to find out just how healthy he was at that moment.

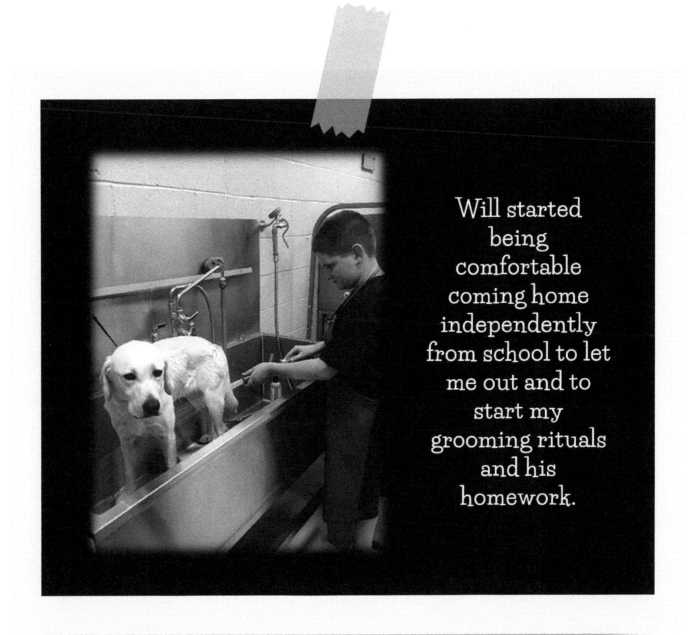

Will started being comfortable coming home independently from school to let me out and to start my grooming rituals and his homework.

Will had appointments with all the special people on his team, which included lots of teachers and doctors, and of course his friends and classmates. Together, with time, treatment, and especially lots of cuddles and licks, Will got better and better.

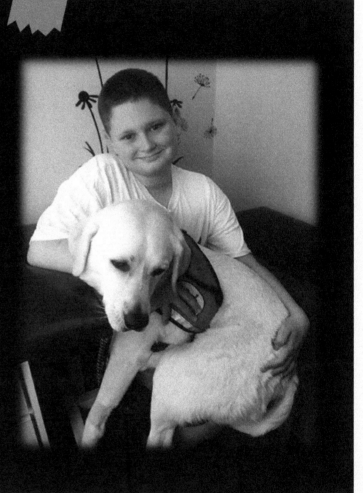

Life with Will still moves fast. My busy boy, Will, has become a better student, a better artist, a better drummer with his school band, an actor in the school shows, and a better gamer with a healthier diet and exercise routine.

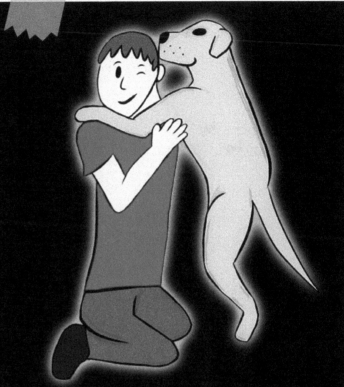

Will is now 17-years-old and we just celebrated our fifth anniversary together.

Will's mom always said my boy, Will, was God's Will, and that he had a big important job to do. She said he was a pioneer in his community - that's someone who is the first to experience something and to teach others about it. Since Will was diagnosed with PANS 11 years ago and treated for what is now is known as autoimmune encephalopathy (say that five times fast!), there were many children who also got the right diagnosis and treatment, too.

autoimmune encephalopathy

autoimmune encephalopathy

autoimmune encephalopathy

autoimmune encephalopathy

autoimmune encephalopathy

When they see us together people often ask
why a boy as tall, and smart, and kind as Will
has a service dog. Will tells them about PANS
and he tells them about me. He says I made
his life better because now he is so much
more healthy and independent.
But I know I won the service dog lottery.
I get to live life with the greatest human ever.

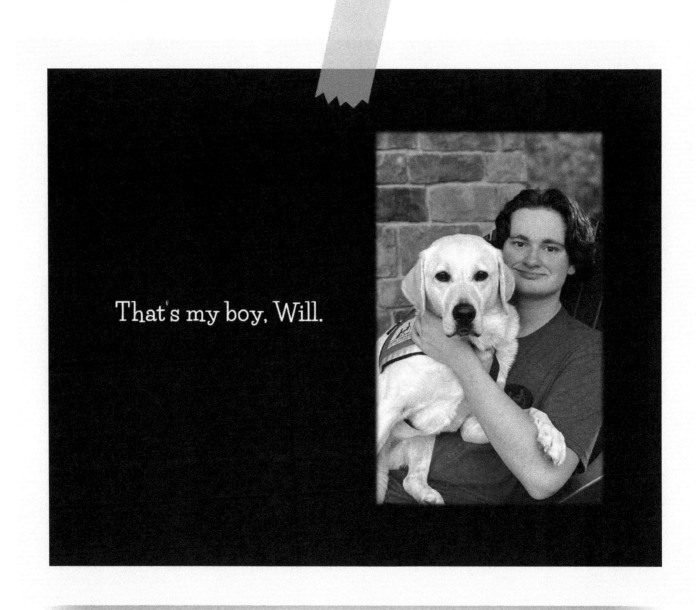

That's my boy, Will.

Canine Companions

Founded in 1975, Canine Companions® is a non-profit organization that enhances the lives of people with disabilities by providing highly trained assistance dogs to people with disabilities and ongoing support to ensure quality partnerships throughout the working life of the dogs.

The assistance dogs Canine Companions breeds, raises, and trains are not just the ears, hands, and legs of their human partners. They're also goodwill ambassadors and often, their best friends. They open up new opportunities and new possibilities, and spread incredible joy. Canine Companions unites people with dogs in a powerful program that leads to greater independence and confidence.

Canine Companions provides assistance dogs for adults with disabilities, people with hearing impairment, wounded and disabled veterans, and working professionals who are matched with assistance dogs in health care, criminal justice, or educational settings. Canine Companions also provides assistance dogs to perform physical tasks for children with a range of disabilities to increase independence with support from an adult handler, usually the child's parent. These extra special dogs like Toshi are called Skilled Companions.

Please visit **www.canine.org** to learn more about these canine angels and how to support the cause.

PANS

PANS, or Pediatric Acute-Onset Neuropsychiatric Syndrome, is the severe and drastic onset of neuropsychiatric symptoms, including anxiety, obsessions, compulsions, emotional lability, depression, irritability, aggression, oppositional behaviors, developmental regression, deterioration in school performance, motor or sensory abnormalities, sleep disturbance, and urinary frequency or enuresis.

PANS is a form of autoimmune encephalopathy or neuroinflammatory disease. Researchers believe that simultaneous exposure to multiple infections and metabolic disturbance disrupt the natural immunological mechanisms that prevent the immune system from attacking self-antigen, and produce an abnormal activation of the immune system that then attacks the cells of the brain. It is believed that some children are predisposed to these dysregulated immune responses.

To learn more about PANS and autoimmune encephalopathy, please visit
www.pandasnetwork.org

CPSIA information can be obtained
at www.ICGtesting.com
Printed in the USA
BVHW021414211221
624588BV00009B/512